WOMEN REPRODUCTIVE HEALTH: ENDOMETRIOSIS, PCOS, OVARIAN CYSTS, UTERINE FIBROIDS, DYSMENORRHEA, AND AMENORRHEA TREATMENT - THE HORMONE REPAIR MANUAL

CONTENTS

Title Page

Copyright

Chapter 1: My fiancée became unwell 1

Chapter 2: My fiancée got admitted to the hospital 5

Chapter 3: My fiancée got diagnosed with pelvic inflammatory disease (PID) and ovarian cysts 8

Chapter 4: Search for alternative treatment approaches 12

Chapter 5: Connection between PID and hormonal imbalance 16

Chapter 6: Effect of hormonal imbalance on endometriosis 20

Chapter 7: Hormonal imbalance EFFECT on polycystic ovary syndrome 24

Chapter 8: Effect of hormonal imbalance on ovarian cysts 28

Chapter 9: Hormonal imbalance EFFECT on uterine fibroids 32

Chapter 10: Effect of hormonal imbalance on menstruation disorders 35

Chapter 11: Natural remedies for hormonal imbalance 39

About The Author 61

Books By This Author 63

CHAPTER 1: MY FIANCÉE BECAME UNWELL

The health of you, your partner, or close family member can really change your life in ways that you never expected. One minute, you could be making plans to work hard and save some money so you can finally invest in your business dream, go to that long awaited vacation, start a family, or buy a home; and the next minute, you are booking appointments with different healthcare professionals, queuing in waiting rooms to see doctors, and setting up reminders so you don't forget to take your medication. I learnt this life lesson the hardest possible way!

It all started on the new year period of 2023. My fiancée and I were all psyched up for the year ahead, making all kinds of work, life, and financial resolutions. Things had seemed pretty good for the previous year (2022), because we had managed to secure a better paying job, a fairly cheap and private housing arrangement, a bike, and two lovely puppies. We were almost 100% sure that the next year would turn out to be same, if not better, for us. We were already making grand plans of upgrading from a bike to a car, building our own home, and finally starting a family. In my head, I was already seeing myself in our new and lovely home while rocking our newborn baby into sleep in my arms as my fiancée is preparing us a nicely cooked meal in the kitchen.

Just as we were settling down to kick off the year, my partner started complaining of random pelvic discomforts and pains. At first, we assumed that maybe it is menstrual cramps, because she usually has one of those rough menstrual periods. So, we decided to give it some time, and observe how it goes. Soon after, she started noticing a unusually smelly and yellowish discharge. Now, we were at a point where we were starting to get worried, and so, we agreed that maybe it was time to see the doctor.

My partner has never once wanted to leave me behind when she is going for doctor appointments. She always wants me by her side to crack her up with my silly jokes so she doesn't have to wait nervously for her turn to see the doctor. Also, believe it or not, she sometimes forgets to describe all her symptoms to the doctor when consulting, and so, she usually wants me there to remind her that when she forgets to mention something. Then, who wouldn't want a comforting hand holding you when you're receiving that scary report from the doctor about what is wrong with your body?

So, when my partner went for the doctor appointment, as usual, she tagged me along. Fortunately, we had set up our healthcare insurance therefore the costs of getting checked up and treated we not really stressing us up. When it was her turn to see the doctor, she described her symptoms and the doctor sent her to the laboratory to provide some samples for testing. The results came back, and luckily, according to the doctor, there wasn't any big problem that some medication couldn't treat. She was diagnosed with a Urinary Tract Infection (UTI) and given some medication before we were sent on our way. After medicating for 2 weeks as per the dosage that had been prescribed, the symptoms my fiancée had been experiencing disappeared. Finally, her usually glowing and smiley personality started coming back. I heaved a sigh of relief at the thought that this harrowing ordeal was finally coming to an end, and now it was time to go back to planning for our bright future.

Turns out I was awfully wrong, and this experience was not ending but rather just beginning. After about a week of completing her medication, my partner once again started experiencing the same symptoms: random pelvic discomforts and abnormally smelly and yellowish discharge. We once more had to rush to the doctor to find out why the medication had not worked as the doctor had promised it would. The doctor told us that the infection had turned out to be resistant to the antibiotics he had prescribed, and thus, he had to prescribe a different set of medications that included stronger and more effective antibiotics that would finish off the infection for once and for all. We went back home, and my fiancée faithfully took her daily dosage with the hope that it would work and allow her to fully recover. Guess what? This time round, the symptoms didn't even subside! She completed her entire prescription while still experiencing pelvic discomforts and an abnormally smelly and yellowish discharge. We earned ourselves another trip to the doctor's office.

CHAPTER 2: MY FIANCÉE GOT ADMITTED TO THE HOSPITAL

The doctor, who happened to be a general practitioner, informed us that there might be an underlying condition that required a more intensive medication approach. The solution? My fiancée would have to be admitted for a week to receive intravenous (IV) injections while being monitored by healthcare professionals. For somebody that had gotten so used to cuddling beside their soulmate the entire night for three straight years, this information felt like someone had dropped a bombshell on me. I immediately started wondering how I was going to survive at home alone for a week without my partner. How was I going to sleep alone on a bed that was meant for two? How was I going to watch movies after a long tiring day without anybody to laugh with when witty remarks are made? Being as scatterbrained as I am, how was I going to find keys and my phone in the house without my fiancée? Regardless, the doctor had said that hospital admission was the only option for us, so there was nothing I could to about it other than oblige.

When leaving the house that morning, we didn't have the slightest idea that my partner would end up being admitted, and so, we were totally unprepared. I had to leave her behind getting admitted while I rushed home to get her some essentials. And unfortunately, we didn't have anybody that could take care of our puppies while my fiancée was admitted at the hospital, thus, after bringing back the essentials I was forced to leave her alone at the hospital and go back home to look after the puppies. Thus, my new routine became waking up early in the morning to go to the hospital and keep my partner company for the whole day, then, heading back home in the evening to take care of our puppies.

Although long and agonizing, the 1-week period my fiancé was supposed to be hospitalized came to an end and she finally got discharged. I escorted her back home with my fingers crossed that this was the last time we were coming to the hospital concerning the pestering and persistent infection that my partner had. But, fate had other plans in mind. The pelvic pain and yellowish discharge symptoms recurred, which forced us to take a fourth trip to the doctor's office. We were at the point where we could no longer withstand the thought of going to see the doctor nor the sight of the seats in the waiting room at the doctor's office. I was getting exasperated and overwhelmed with thoughts, wondering when this saddening experience was going to end. As we waited at the doctor's lounge for our turn to see him, my fiancée looked at me with a sad expression, and said, "I really hope I won't be getting admitted this time round. I can't stand the pain of the intravenous catheter getting inserted into my arm nor the discomfort of living with it for an entire week. I can't stomach the taste of the hospital meals or sleeping on the hospital bed for the entire night."

CHAPTER 3: MY FIANCÉE GOT DIAGNOSED WITH PELVIC INFLAMMATORY DISEASE (PID) AND OVARIAN CYSTS

When it was our turn to consult, the general practitioner told us that the infection was becoming resistant. Thus, the next option was booking an appointment with a specialist doctor - a gynecologist. As fate would have it, the healthcare facility didn't have an in-house specialist doctor, and therefore, my fiancée had to be admitted as we waited for the available gynecologist to do hospital rounds. The general practitioner also advised my partner to go for an ultrasound scan at the sonographer which would help in determining the exact cause of the symptoms being experienced. The ultrasound scan indicated that the UTI my fiancée had been diagnosed with had developed into a pelvic inflammatory disease (PID). The sonographer also noted that she had developed some ovarian cysts, but they were of a small size. We were advised to wait out the ovarian cysts and see it they would disappear naturally since they were small. Thus, the treatment approach shifted from focusing on the UTI to focusing on the PID.

When my fiancée finally consulted with the gynecologist, she was advised to proceed with the PID medication that was being received intravenously while being observed by the healthcare professionals. My partner was also told that she would experience some fertility and conception issues so long as she was still diagnosed with the ovarian cysts and PID. At this point, she started getting depressed because our dream of starting a family together was being threatened at the core. She couldn't withstand the idea of not being able to give birth because of a simple infection that had started out as a normal UTI.

But, I stood by her side and tried as best as I could to look strong for her. I encouraged her with the thought that there is no infinite experience to life, and that, everything that has a beginning always has an ending to it. All we had to do was persevere and hold on as we wait to rejoice at the end of our harrowing experience. And, although hopelessly, my partner managed to push on and fight as hard as she could.

One week after getting admitted, my fiancée finally finished her prescription for intravenous injections and got discharged from the hospital. The symptoms had disappeared, and we were hopeful that maybe she had fully healed this time round. We were hopeful that maybe there wouldn't be a next time in regards to visiting the doctor's office for consultation about the infection.

But, as you might have guessed already, fate had other plans in store for us. Two weeks after being discharged, my fiancée once again started experiencing the pelvic pain and yellowish discharge symptoms. This time round we booked an appointment with a gynecologist, who told us that the PID was not responding to medication because of the ovarian cysts. Thus, my partner would have to go into surgery to remove the ovarian cysts before she is treated for the PID. And apparently, the surgical procedure had a very high probability of leading to infertility for life. Since my fiancée wanted a baby more than anything else in this world, we became stuck at crossroads. She did want to get healed for once and for all, but not if it came at the cost of our dream to start a family together. Therefore, we decided to postpone the surgery and seek different opinions from other sources before ultimately sealing our fate.

CHAPTER 4: SEARCH FOR ALTERNATIVE TREATMENT APPROACHES

At this point, I suggested to my fiancée to look for other individuals going through the same ordeal she was experiencing so as to determine how they had dealt with the infection, and whether they had managed to heal fully. She went to social media platforms such as Reddit, Telegram, and Facebook to look for women forums and communities or rather groups that were dedicated to the healthcare of women's reproductive system. Unfortunately, there were none dedicated to women experiencing PID and ovarian cysts at the same time. Thus, she was forced to post in other random female forums and communities asking anybody who had been diagnosed with PID or ovarian cysts to send a private message for further communication. Believe it or not, her inbox was flooded with messages from other women suffering from a plight similar to hers.

Some had PID that was resistant to antibiotics, others had large ovarian cysts, while other had both PID and ovarian cysts like my fiancée. She decided to form a WhatsApp group to enable them share their experiences and inform each other about updates in their treatment. Unfortunately, none of the women had managed to heal fully from their PID. They would get treated, then the symptoms disappear for some time before recurring. Rather than get a solution to the problem, and hope of recovering, we ended up learning that overcoming this challenge was going to be an uphill task since some of the women had been struggling with the PID for as long as 2 years, with no cure in sight.

Eventually, my fiancée was advised by her friend, who was a nurse practitioner, to do a culture and sensitivity test to determine the exact bacteria that had infected her, and the antibiotics that would effectively treat the medical condition. And so, we went for the test and she was given a new prescription. When she finished her dosage, the symptoms cleared, and we decided to go for an ultrasound to determine whether the infection had been treated fully. The sonographer told us that the infection had cleared out, and the ovarian cysts had also disappeared. We finally managed to be happy and stress-free for the first time in a period of over 2 months. My fiancée had managed to treat the PID without having to go for surgery and risking the likelihood of us starting a family together. It was now time to get back to building our life.

Or so we thought! Unfortunately, when she went through her menstrual periods, the pelvic pain and yellowish discharge symptoms started to recur. She once more went for a culture and sensitivity test and was given an additional prescription that would last for a week. This time round, the medication given after performing the culture and sensitivity test would effectively finish off the infection. But, each time my fiancée went through her menstrual periods, the infection would come back. We were at a point where the doctors were beginning to wonder what could be the problem. They couldn't understand why the PID kept healing and reappearing every time. To make matters worse, the doctors suggested that the infection could be recurring due to unprotected sex with numerous partners. This information actually led to the occurrence of trust issues in our relationship because we were suspicious of each other. The trust issues and suspicions got so bad that we started having arguments accusing each other of infidelity.

CHAPTER 5: CONNECTION BETWEEN PID AND HORMONAL IMBALANCE

However, I had more faith in us, and thus, I decided to set aside the thoughts of infidelity that were planted by the doctor's suggestions. I decided to do some research to find out what could be the problem. I particularly was focused on the trend we had identified - the PID kept recurring after my fiancée had gone through her menstrual periods. I managed to learn that, under normal circumstances, the pH value of the vagina is supposed to be around 4.0, which is somewhat acidic (Clarke et al., 2012). This acidic environment is vital and fundamental for the vaginal flora because the acidity helps to balance out the state of good and bad bacteria in the female reproductive system.

But, during menstrual periods, there is production of blood discharge in large quantities, and blood generally has a pH value of around 7.0, which is considerably alkaline. Thus, the blood discharge produced during menstrual periods generally increases the pH of the vagina, which upsets the optimal environment for balancing of vaginal flora (Farage et al., 2010).

But, under normal circumstances, the progesterone hormone helps to correct the pH value of the vagina after the menstruation periods since it is slightly acidic. The progesterone hormone is generally produced during the second phase of the menstrual cycle that is otherwise referred to as the luteal phase. This particular phase comes before menstruation and after ovulation whereby the remnants of the ovarian follicle, after the ovule has been formed, transform into corpus luteum that produces progesterone (Hamidovic et al., 2020).

Since my partner's PID kept recurring after she had undergone her menstrual periods, I deduced that the menstruation was occurring, and thus, upsetting the pH value of the vagina. Then, there wasn't sufficient production of the progesterone hormone to help regulate the pH of the vagina after the blood discharge produced during menstruation increases it (Song et al., 2020). Thus, the state of bad and good bacteria in the vagina would become unbalanced with the bad bacteria outgrowing the good bacteria, which led to the occurrence of the PID.

The low levels of the progesterone hormone had occurred because of preceding low levels of the estrogen hormone. The estrogen hormone is in charge of increasing production of the luteinizing hormone that in turn motivates the ovarian follicle to release an egg before turning into the corpus luteum that produces progesterone. Thus, low levels of the estrogen hormone can result in failure to ovulate and subsequent failure to form corpus luteum that should produce the progesterone hormone.

Therefore, my fiancée had an issue of hormonal imbalance which was consequently causing an infection. And, when we were going to the doctor, they were only treating the PID, which was a reaction of the hormonal imbalance while doing nothing about the underlying issue. That is why the infection kept recurring no matter how much it was getting treated.

CHAPTER 6: EFFECT OF HORMONAL IMBALANCE ON ENDOMETRIOSIS

I did further research on the issue of hormonal balance and discovered that it is very important in the female reproductive system, and any changes can lead to some significant healthcare issues (Cheng et al., 2022). Case in point, hormonal imbalance can lead to the medical condition otherwise referred to as endometriosis. This healthcare issue is generally caused by the growth of endometrium, body tissues that are considerably similar to the uterus lining, in areas such as ovaries, fallopian tube, and outer parts of the uterus (Raja et al., 2021). Under normal circumstances, the endometrium is produced during the menstruation cycle to enable a fertilized egg in implantation and subsequent development into an embryo when conception occurs. However, the endometrium is shed during menstruation if conception fails to occur.

The endometriosis tissue is generally sensitive to the estrogen hormone in that this particular hormone promotes its growth and development. Thus, high levels of the estrogen hormone can lead to an overgrowth of the endometriosis tissue in areas such as ovaries, fallopian tube, and outer parts of the uterus (Smolarz et al., 2021). Estrogen levels tend to be particularly high some days before or during menstruation periods. And hence, the growth of the endometriosis tissue can be accelerated during this time frame. This commonly leads to severe endometriosis symptoms during menstruation periods. The symptoms in question include but are not limited to menstrual disorders, painful sex, pelvic pain, and inflammation or scarring of the reproductive system (Alimdjanovna, 2021).

In some extreme cases, endometriosis has been known to cause fertility issues in women. This is because the excessive growth of endometrial tissue cause distortion of the female reproductive system by creating cysts, adhesions, and scar tissue, which prevent effective meeting of sperm and eggs (Sharma and Tripathi, 2022). Also, the growth of endometrial tissue outside the uterus causes inflammation, and the production of inflammatory substances have an undermining effect on the uterus, ovaries, and fallopian tube, which reduces the probability of conception occurring. Besides, endometrial tissue, as we have ascertained above, have an undermining effect in the uterus. Thus, endometriosis can negatively affect the receptivity of the endometrium to implantation of the embryo, which reduces the likelihood of fertilized eggs attaching and developing (Pirtea et al., 2023).

According to the World Health Organization (WHO), the endometriosis healthcare complication affects over 190 million females in the world (WHO, 2023b). The figure mentioned above translates to about 10% of the women and girls that are within the reproductive age bracket. To make matters worse, pharmaceutical companies and scientists are yet to discover an effective cure for endometriosis (Smolarz et al., 2021). Thus, the currently prevailing treatment approaches for this medical condition focus on treatment and management of the symptoms. Due to this fact, it is essential that endometriosis is diagnosed in its early stages to ensure effective treatment.

CHAPTER 7: HORMONAL IMBALANCE EFFECT ON POLYCYSTIC OVARY SYNDROME

Other than endometriosis, hormonal imbalance has been associated with the medical condition of polycystic ovary syndrome (PCOS) that generally affects women and girls. PCOS occurs in females when there are significantly high production rates of male hormones such as testosterone, that are otherwise referred to as androgens (Khan et al., 2019). Testosterone, among other androgens, are produced by the ovarian follicles during the middle of the menstruation cycle, after they have been stimulated by the luteinizing hormone (LH). Thus, excessive production of LH can consequently lead to high production levels of androgens such as testosterone (Dinsdale and Crespi, 2021). The production of the LH, on the other hand, is regulated by estrogen through negative feedback. Therefore, high levels of estrogen hormone can lead to excessive production of LH, which in turn causes production of high levels of androgens such as testosterone.

Under normal circumstances, androgens play fundamental roles in the female body. For instance, they facilitate muscle growth and development in females in addition to helping the maintenance of optimal bone density. Also, from a reproductive perspective, androgens are essential in the regulation of the ovulation process as well as sexual libido in females (Bianchi et al., 2021). When in excess, androgens are generally converted into progesterone and estrogen hormones. For example, the testosterone hormone is converted into the estrogen hormone in adipose tissue as well as ovaries with the help of the aromatase enzyme (Shah and Shrivastava, 2023). The process mentioned above is made possible by the aromatase enzyme catalyzing the conversion of testosterone molecules into estrogen molecules through addition of aromatic ring structure to the androgen molecule. The estrogen hormone regulates the process above, which is otherwise referred to as aromatization, through negative feedback. Thus, low levels of the estrogen undermine the capacity of the female reproductive system to regulate conversion of the testosterone hormone into the estrogen hormone (Xu and Qiao, 2022).

PCOS is characterized by numerous signs and symptoms. The most physical symptom of PCOS is growth of excessive hair on a female, a condition that is otherwise referred to as hirsutism (Spritzer et al., 2022). Besides, PCOS can result in acne formation and menstruation disorders, whereby an individual skips some menstruation periods or the periods occur irregularly, and in some extreme cases there is no ovulation (Purwar and Nagpure, 2022). Also, PCOS can undermine the metabolism rates in females whereby it causes insulin resistance, a condition that can consequently result in an increased probability of being diagnosed with type 2 diabetes, obesity, and/ or high blood pressure (Xu and Qiao, 2022). PCOS can further lead to fertility issues in females because the underlying issue of hormonal imbalance undermines the process of ovulation.

According to a report by the World Health Organisation, PCOS affects approximately 116 million reproductive-aged females globally. The prevalence of PCOS has also been realised to be higher among some ethnicities and these populations tend to experience severe complications related to metabolic problems (Jabeen et al., 2022). As if that is not bad enough, there is no definite cure for PCOS. However, associated comorbidities can be addressed to improve symptoms, quality of life, and minimise the long-term complications that result from PCOS (WHO, 2023a). Therefore, certain symptoms can be minimised through changes in lifestyle, birth control medicines, and surgery to stimulate regular ovulation.

CHAPTER 8: EFFECT OF HORMONAL IMBALANCE ON OVARIAN CYSTS

Hormonal imbalance can additionally result in the occurrence of ovarian cysts in women and girls that are of a reproductive age (Farkas et al., 2023). Ovarian cysts are sacs filled with fluid that generally form in ovaries and they can be either functional, which implies they are a normal part of the menstruation cycle, or pathological. Ovarian cysts occur via two main processes, whereby the first process is facilitated after an ovarian follicle develops but fails to undergo the process of ovulation to release an egg for fertilization (NHS, 2023). In this particular instance, the ovarian follicle will develop into a follicular cyst.

The second process of cyst formation in the ovary occurs after the ovarian follicle has released an egg for fertilization (Woldemeskel, 2022). The follicle should then transform into a structure that is commonly referred to as the corpus luteum, which produces the progesterone hormone before dissolving. If the corpus luteum fails to dissolve effectively, it can lead to the formation of a corpus luteum cyst.

Both of the processes mentioned above are generally regulated by a hormone otherwise referred to as Luteinizing Hormone (LH) whereby an increase in its levels often signal the ovarian follicle to rupture and release an egg, a procedure called ovulation (Oduwole et al., 2021). Conversely, a decrease in the LH often leads to minimized functionality within the corpus luteum, and thus it ends up dissolving (Przygrodzka et al., 2021). On the other hand, LH, as previously mentioned, is generally controlled by the estrogen hormone in that an increase in the latter leads to a surge in the initial and vice versa (Nedresky and Singh, 2019).

In most cases, ovarian cysts tend to be asymptomatic, but when the signs and symptoms manifest they could include: a pelvic pain that ranges from a dull ache to sharp and severe on one or both sides of the pelvis or abdomen, menstruation disorders, frequent urination, nausea and/or vomiting, and difficulty emptying bowels.

The prevalence of ovarian cysts has been reported to range between 8% and 18% of premenopausal and postmenopausal women respectively. A significant number of post-menopausal cysts have been realised to be persistent for years. And this is despite that fact, the treatment options for ovarian cysts are many. Regardless, the ultimate management is dependent on the menopausal status, age of the patient, size of the cyst, and if the cyst indicates malignancy characteristics (Mobeen and Apostol, 2020).

It is important to note that, unilocular cysts, which are less than 10 cm, are often benign regardless of the age of the patient. This implies that the patient can be asymptomatic and can therefore only be monitored using serial transvaginal ultrasound. And, in case a cyst does not resolve after several menstrual cycles, it implies that it is not a functional cyst, thus further workup is required, which in most instances is surgical intervention.

CHAPTER 9: HORMONAL IMBALANCE EFFECT ON UTERINE FIBROIDS

Besides, hormonal imbalance can lead to a female reproductive condition commonly known as uterine fibroids, leiomyomas, or myomas (Giuliani et al., 2020). This condition primarily involves the development of noncancerous growths within the uterus often within the childbearing age bracket. The growths in question tend to vary in size from seed-like sizes to huge masses that distort the uterus shape.

Uterine fibroids generally have estrogen hormone receptors, and thus, they tend to have high sensitivity and responsiveness to the said hormone. When the uterine fibroid receptors and estrogen hormone bind, the growth rates of the fibroids is stimulated significantly. If has been noted within the medical field that the occurrence of uterine fibroids therefore varies with the levels of the estrogen hormone within the body (Alsudairi et al., 2021). Case in point, during the reproductive years of a female, estrogen production is high and thus uterine fibroids are encouraged to grow but when menopause approaches estrogen hormone reduces, and thus, uterine fibroids reduce and/or stop growing.

As previously mentioned, uterine fibroids are generally benign, and thus, there is a considerably minimal probability of uterine cancer occurring as a result of these growths (Patel et al., 2023). However, the fibroids tend to cause numerous symptoms and signs, which include but are not limited to: menstruation disorders, pelvic pain or pressure, frequent urination, and backaches.

Uterine fibroids have a recorded prevalence of up to 68.6% (Lou et al., 2023). Over the past three decades, the prevalent cases of uterine fibroids have risen steadily from 126.41 million to 226.05 million cases globally, indicating a 78.82% growth. To treat uterine fibroids, healthcare professionals may recommend embolization, a minimally invasive procedure often performed on an outpatient basis. Uterine fibroids embolization entails cutting off the supply of blood to the fibroids, which causes their shrinking. Also, hysterectomy, a medical procedure to remove the uterus, can be performed (Liu et al., 2023). This method is regarded as the major treatment for uterine fibroids as it tends to present a 100% surety of the fibroids not recurring. Hysterectomy is usually reserved for females with extremely heavy bleeding and are approaching or post-menopause, and have enormous uterine fibroids.

CHAPTER 10: EFFECT OF HORMONAL IMBALANCE ON MENSTRUATION DISORDERS

Last, hormonal imbalance has generally been associated with various menstruation disorders. I will categorize the said disorders into two classes depending on their major defining symptoms and signs. For instance, metrorrhagia, hypomenorrhea, menorrhagia, amenorrhea, and oligomenorrhea all relate to the process of blood discharge during menstruation periods. This is evident in that metrorrhagia involves irregular blood discharge in between normal menstrual periods and menorrhagia is the occurrence of excessive blood discharge during menstrual periods (Jarzabek-Bielecka et al., 2019; Mohammed, 2022). The two menstruation disorders mentioned above are generally caused by the excessive production of estrogen hormone. This hormone, as we have already determined above, tends to cause a reaction of the uterine lining that has estrogen receptors. Thus, whenever its produced in high levels it leads to the overgrowth and thickening of the uterine lining). When the uterine lining undergoes shedding during the menstrual period, it subsequently causes heavier and prolonged blood discharge or irregular bleeding between normal menstrual periods.

Conversely, hypomenorrhea is a condition characterized by considerably scanty or light menstruation periods, oligomenorrhea involves the occurrence of irregular or infrequent menstruation periods, and amenorrhea is the lack of menstruation periods (Rahmadani and Furqan, 2022). All of the three menstruation disorders mentioned above are generally caused by production of insufficient levels of the estrogen hormone. This is because low estrogen levels affect the optimal growth of the uterine lining during the menstruation cycle, and thus, when the uterine lining is shed, the blood discharge observed is minimal or non-existent.

The second class of menstruation disorders entails dysmenorrhea, which is a medical term that refers to the occurrence of menstruation periods that cause physical pain or discomfort that ranges from mild to extreme or severe (McKenna and Fogleman, 2021). The physical pain manifests as a result of muscle contractions referred to as cramps that are caused by lipid compounds known as prostaglandins. The lipid compounds mentioned previously are usually produced within the uterine lining or endometrium during the menstruation cycle (Lee et al., 2020). The production rates of prostaglandins generally increase in preparing for the shedding of the uterine lining during menstruation periods. This is because the muscle contractions they cause are required in order to expel the shed uterine lining among other uterus tissue and menstrual blood.

The production of prostaglandins is often regulated by the estrogen hormone. This is because estrogen hormone levels hike during the menstruation cycle consequently leading to the stimulation of the uterine lining to produce more prostaglandins (Palter et al., 2002). Thus, significantly high levels of the estrogen hormone cause high production rates of prostaglandins, which cause stronger muscle contractions, and hence dysmenorrhea.

Menstruation disorders are one of the most occurring gynaecologic problems affecting females of child bearing age. They have a global prevalence of 75%, hence the most frequent reasons for women consulting physicians (Igbokwe et al., 2021). There are however various ways to treat menstruation disorders. These include: Nonsteroidal anti-inflammatory drugs (NSAIDs) such as ibuprofen and naproxen, and Acetaminophen, which aid in relieving cramps pain. In addition, oral contraceptives aid in reducing heavy bleeding and regulating menstrual periods. Also, the LNG-IUS (Mirena), which is a progesterone intrauterine device (IUD), is oftentimes recommended as the first treatment for heavy bleeding. Furthermore, endometrial ablation, a surgical option that destroys the uterine lining, is recommended for females with heavy menstrual flow, as it helps in reducing the menstrual flow. It is important to note that in cases whereby medical therapy is unsuccessful, hysterectomy may be considered.

CHAPTER 11: NATURAL REMEDIES FOR HORMONAL IMBALANCE

Overall, I determined that the estrogen hormone is one of the most fundamental hormones within the female body in general, and the female reproductive system specifically. Thus, any hormonal imbalances that impact the optimal levels of the estrogen hormone can result in numerous medical conditions. For instance, when estrogen hormone levels are high, healthcare issues such as Polycystic Ovary Syndrome (PCOS), endometriosis, uterine fibroids, ovarian cysts, and some menstrual disorders manifest. Contrarily, when estrogen hormone levels are low, medical conditions like Pelvic Inflammatory Disease (PID), ovarian cysts, and some menstrual disorders start occurring.

Most healthcare professionals often advise patients to perform the hormonal replacement therapy (HRT) once the issue of hormonal imbalance occurs. HRT can thus by extension treat some of the medical conditions I have discussed above or relieve their symptoms. The process of HRT is mostly achieved with the aid of synthetic hormones in healthcare facilities. For instance, if the HRT procedure is focused on the estrogen hormone, synthetic steroid estrogens such as ethinyl estradiol, estradiol valerate, estropipate, conjugate esterified estrogen, or quinestrol (Delgado and Lopez-Ojeda, 2023). However, the use of synthetic steroid estrogens presents some significant medical risks. Case in point, pre-existing research attempts have determined that long-term usage of synthetic steroid estrogens can lead to an increased risk of breast cancer. Also, initiating the HRT procedure after midlife stage significantly increases the risk of dementia occurring. Besides, if you are utilizing synthetic steroid estrogens with the uterus still present and intact without progestin – a synthetic progesterone hormone, there is a higher likelihood of endometrial cancer manifesting (Cleveland Clinic, 2021). Last, there is reason to believe that application of synthetic steroid estrogens sometimes leads to blood clots and thus there is a high likelihood of stroke occurring. Thus, HRT using synthetic hormones is more or less being stuck between the devil and the deep blue sea.

But, there is a more tolerable alternative if you don't want to treat one medical issue while creating the ground for another healthcare complication in the future. Fortunately, some of the food we eat on a daily basis does not only serve to address our nutritional needs, but can also replenish the lacking components of the human body in addition to correcting certain health issues. Hence, you can use a more natural based approach of HRT that is based on different foodstuffs. This is because humans are not the only mammals that produce estrogen, as cows and goats can also generate this particular hormone (Malekinejad and Rezabakhsh, 2015). Thus, consuming milk and dairy products or meat can result in the absorption of the estrogen hormone produced by animals.

Besides, there is a naturally produced plant element

that functions in a manner that is similar to the estrogen produced by the human body. The plant compound in question is referred to as phytoestrogens or dietary estrogen, and it has a chemical structure that resembles that of estrogen, which allows it to mimic actions of the said hormone (Berkheiser, 2023). For instance, phytoestrogens can essentially attach themselves to the receptors for the estrogen hormone existing within human cells thus affecting the normal estrogen functions throughout the human body (Kuiper et al., 1998).

Phytoestrogens can be divided into three further categories: lignans, resveratrol, and flavonoids (WebMD, 2022). Under the lignans category, there are numerous foodstuffs that contain phytoestrogens, but seeds such as flaxseeds and sesame seeds have the highest content since there are close to 300 milligrams of lignans for each 100 grams of these seeds (Rodriguez-Garcia et al., 2019). Whole grains such as wheat, buckwheat, barley, millet, rye, and oats; nuts such as peanuts, walnuts, hazelnuts, macadamias, pistachios, and cashew nuts are also high in lignans, especially within the bran layer. Finally, there is reason to believe that coffee and tea contain some significant levels of lignans (Peterson et al., 2010).

Conversely, under the resveratrol category, there are numerous foodstuffs that contain phytoestrogens, but grapes have the highest content since resveratrol accounts for about 5 to 10% of the biomass within the grape fruit skin (Rocha-Gonzalenz et al., 2008). As a result, most of the contemporary grape juices and wine have a concentration of resveratrol that ranges from 0.05 to 25 milligrams per liter. You can also expect to find resveratrol in foods such as cocoa, chocolate, blueberries, bilberries, and cranberries (Oregon State University, n.d.).

Finally, under the flavonoids category of phytoestrogens, there are further sub-categories, but the most significant are the isoflavones in regards to the quantity of phytoestrogens. The isoflavones sub-category of flavonoids generally contains legumes such as beans, peas, and lentils. But, soybeans are the isoflavones with the highest phytoestrogens content (Gacek, 2014). Evidence suggests that there are approximately 3.5 milligrams of phytoestrogens in each gram of soybeans (Messina, 2016).

If you have some of the healthcare issues such as menstrual disorders, ovarian cysts, and PID that occur as a result of low levels of the estrogen hormone, and you want to start your journey into achieving hormonal balance with natural remedies such as dieting, I have go you covered. Based on the information provided above, my fiancée and I created a meal plan that majorly contains foods rich in phytoestrogens. The diet plan is provided here:

7-day diet plan for healing hormonal imbalance

Day 1:

Breakfast: Oatmeal topped with blueberries and flaxseeds.

Snack: Greek yogurt with a handful of mixed nuts.

Lunch: Lentil and vegetable soup.

Snack: Sliced cucumbers with hummus.

Dinner: Grilled chicken breast with quinoa and steamed broccoli.

Day 2:

Breakfast: Whole-grain toast with peanut butter and sliced banana.

Snack: Mixed berries (cranberries, bilberries, and blueberries).

Lunch: Spinach and walnut salad with vinaigrette dressing.

Snack: Carrot sticks with hummus.

Dinner: Baked salmon with asparagus and a side of brown rice.

Day 3:

Breakfast: Scrambled eggs with spinach and a cup of green tea.

Snack: Handful of mixed nuts.

Lunch: Chickpea salad with a variety of veggies and a tahini dressing.

Snack: Sliced apple with almond butter.

Dinner: Beef stir-fry with broccoli, peppers, and sesame seeds.

Day 4:

Breakfast: Chia seed pudding with sliced strawberries.

Snack: A small serving of dark chocolate.

Lunch: Quinoa and black bean salad.

Snack: Greek yogurt with honey and walnuts.

Dinner: Grilled pork chops with roasted sweet potatoes.

Day 5:

Breakfast: Whole-grain cereal with milk (or a milk substitute) and sliced bananas.

Snack: A handful of grapes.

Lunch: Lentil soup with a side of whole-grain bread

Snack: Sliced cucumber with tzatziki sauce.

Dinner: Baked chicken breast with brown rice and steamed green beans.

Day 6:

Breakfast: Smoothie with soy milk, frozen mixed berries, and a scoop of protein powder.

Snack: Trail mix with a variety of nuts and dried cranberries.

Lunch: Spinach and feta stuffed chicken breast.

Snack: Sliced pear with cottage cheese.

Dinner: Grilled goat meat with quinoa and roasted zucchini.

Day 7:

Breakfast: Scrambled tofu with spinach and a cup of coffee.

Snack: A piece of dark chocolate.

Lunch: Split pea soup with a side of whole-grain crackers.

Snack: Sliced bell peppers with peanut butter.

Dinner: Grilled lamb chops with couscous and steamed carrots.

In addition to observing the diet plan above, we made some lifestyle changes to support the process of healing the hormonal imbalance challenge my fiancée was undergoing. For instance, my fiancée had to limit usage of beauty and hair care products such as shampoo and hair conditioner, moisturizers and lotions, and makeup. This is because a significant proportion of the said products have some significant levels of a chemical referred to as parabens, which is considered to have endocrine disrupting properties and can thus cause hormonal imbalance (Nowak et al., 2018; WebMD, 2021).

Also, my fiancée reduced usage of plastics such as cups, plates, and water bottles for purposes of consuming food. This is because most plastics contain a compound referred to as phthalates, which are a class of chemicals aimed at enhancing the durability of plastics (Starkman, 2021; CDC, 2021). There is scientific evidence that suggests phthalates have the capability of disrupting hormonal balance in the human body (Chen et al., 2014). Lastly, my fiancée reduced her levels of alcohol consumption because there is reason to believe that heavy alcoholic consumption can result in hormonal balance issues.(Emanuele et al., 2002).

After three months of religiously following the diet plan above, my fiancée started noticing some pretty amazing results. She started by recording her first week without any abdominal pains. This progressively increased to a month without any abdominal pains, and in no time, she had hit a milestone of 3 months without any abdominal pains. What's more? Six months after we started the dieting plan above, we finally managed to conceive. This was a great turnaround from being faced with the probability of losing the ability to get pregnant while being treated for the PID. If the diet plan above worked wonders for us, it could do some miracles for you too.

By now you might have noticed that I haven't mentioned of natural remedies and dieting plans for healthcare complications such as menstrual disorders, uterine fibroids, endometriosis, PCOS, and ovarian cysts that are caused by high levels of the estrogen hormone. Does that mean there is no natural remedy for those experiencing these medical conditions? Well, no!

Just as there are naturally occurring compounds in plants that act as estrogens - phytoestrogens, there are also some naturally occurring elements in plants that act as anti-estrogens. What does this mean? Well, anti-estrogens basically limit the endocrine glands from overproducing the estrogen hormone in addition to breaking down and excreting the excess levels of the same hormone. And good news is - there are plenty of naturally occurring anti-estrogens that are edible.

Case in point, turmeric, which is often used as a spice, has a compound called curcumin that has been found to particularly reduce production levels of estradiol - the most significant type of the estrogen hormone in women that are yet to hit menopause (Zhang et al., 2013). Also, some mushrooms such as the oyster mushroom and medicinal mushrooms have a compound called hispolon. This element, according to scientific evidence, can be fundamental in regards to reducing the levels of the estrogen hormone. This is because it inhibits the aromatase enzyme that catalyzes the conversion of the testosterone hormone into the estrogen hormone (Kikuchi et al., 2017; Wang et al., 2017). Last, cruciferous vegetables such as kales, broccoli, cauliflower, cabbage, and collard greens have high content of glucobrassicin which can consequently be broken down into Indole-3-carbinol (I3C) that has anti-estrogenic effects (Oregon State University, n.d.).

So, if you have healthcare complications such as menstrual disorders, uterine fibroids, endometriosis, PCOS, and ovarian cysts that are caused by high levels of the estrogen hormone, and you need a natural remedy, all you have to do is eat plenty of turmeric, mushrooms, and cruciferous vegetables.

References

Alimdjanovna, T.N., 2021. Endometriosis: Relevance, clinic and treatment. Asian Journal Of Multidimensional Research, 10(4), pp.438-443.

Alsudairi, H.N., Alrasheed, A.T. and Dvornyk, V., 2021. Estrogens and uterine fibroids: an integrated view. Научные результаты биомедицинских исследований, 7(2), pp.156-163.

Berkheiser, K., 2023. 11 Foods High in Phytestrogens. Healthline, https://www.healthline.com/nutrition/foods-with-estrogen

Bianchi, V.E., Bresciani, E., Meanti, R., Rizzi, L., Omeljaniuk, R.J. and Torsello, A., 2021. The role of androgens in women's health and wellbeing. Pharmacological research, 171, p.105758.

CDC, 2021. Phthalates. Centre for Disease Control and Prevention. https://www.cdc.gov/biomonitoring/Phthalates_FactSheet.html#:~:text=Phthalates%20are%20a%20group%20of,%2C%20shampoos%2C%20hair%20sprays).

Chen, X., Xu, S., Tan, T., Lee, S.T., Cheng, S.H., Lee, F.W.F., Xu, S.J.L. and Ho, K.C., 2014. Toxicity and estrogenic endocrine disrupting activity of phthalates and their mixtures. International journal of environmental research and public health, 11(3), pp.3156-3168.

Cheng, C.H., Chen, L.R. and Chen, K.H., 2022. Osteoporosis due to hormone imbalance: an overview of the effects of estrogen deficiency and glucocorticoid overuse on bone turnover. International Journal of Molecular Sciences, 23(3), p.1376.

Clarke, M.A., Rodriguez, A.C., Gage, J.C., Herrero, R., Hildesheim, A., Wacholder, S., Burk, R. and Schiffman, M., 2012. A large, population-based study of age-related associations between vaginal pH and human papillomavirus infection. BMC infectious diseases, 12(1), p.33.

Dinsdale, N.L. and Crespi, B.J., 2021. Endometriosis and polycystic ovary syndrome are diametric disorders. Evolutionary applications, 14(7), pp.1693-1715.

Emanuele, M.A., Wezeman, F. and Emanuele, N.V., 2002. Alcohol's effects on female reproductive function. Alcohol Research & Health, 26(4), p.274.

Farage, M.A., Miller, K.W. and Sobel, J.D., 2010. Dynamics of the vaginal ecosystem—hormonal influences. Infectious Diseases: Research and Treatment, 3, pp.IDRT-S3903.

Farkas, A.H., Abumusa, H. and Rossiter, B., 2023. Structural gynecological disease: fibroids, endometriosis, ovarian cysts. Medical Clinics, 107(2), pp.317-328.

Gacek, M., 2014. Soy and legume seeds as sources of isoflavones: selected individual determinants of their consumption in a group of perimenopausal women. Menopause Review/ Przegląd Menopauzalny, 13(1), pp.27-31.

Giuliani, E., As-Sanie, S. and Marsh, E.E., 2020. Epidemiology and management of uterine fibroids. International Journal of Gynecology & Obstetrics, 149(1), pp.3-9.

Hamidovic, A., Karapetyan, K., Serdarevic, F., Choi, S.H., Eisenlohr-Moul, T. and Pinna, G., 2020. Higher circulating cortisol in the follicular vs. luteal phase of the menstrual cycle: a meta-analysis. Frontiers in endocrinology, 11, p.311.

Igbokwe, U.C. and John-Akinola, Y.O., 2021. Knowledge of menstrual disorders and health seeking behaviour among female undergraduate students of University of Ibadan, Nigeria. Annals of Ibadan Postgraduate Medicine, 19(1), pp.40-48.

Jabeen, A., Yamini, V., Amberina, A.R., Eshwar, M.D., Vadakedath, S., Begum, G.S. and Kandi, V., 2022. Polycystic Ovarian Syndrome: Prevalence, Predisposing Factors, and Awareness Among Adolescent and Young Girls of South India. Cureus, 14(8).

Jarzabek-Bielecka, G., Mizgier, M. and Kedzia, W., 2019. Metrorrhagia iuvenilis and Premenstrual Syndrome as frequent problems of adolescent gynecology with aspects of diet therapy. Ginekologia Polska, 90(7), pp.423-429.

Khan, M.J., Ullah, A. and Basit, S., 2019. Genetic basis of polycystic ovary syndrome (PCOS): current perspectives. The application of clinical genetics, pp.249-260.

Kikuchi, T., Motoyashiki, N., Yamada, T., Shibatani,

K., Ninomiya, K., Morikawa, T. and Tanaka, R., 2017. Ergostane-type sterols from king trumpet mushroom (Pleurotus eryngii) and their inhibitory effects on aromatase. International journal of molecular sciences, 18(11), p.2479.

Kuiper, G.G., Lemmen, J.G., Carlsson, B.O., Corton, J.C., Safe, S.H., Van Der Saag, P.T., Van Der Burg, B. and Gustafsson, J.A., 1998. Interaction of estrogenic chemicals and phytestrogens with estrogen receptor β. Endocrinology, 139(10), pp.4252-4263.

Lee, K., Lee, S.H. and Kim, T.H., 2020. The biology of prostaglandins and their role as a target for allergic airway disease therapy. International journal of molecular sciences, 21(5), p.1851.

Liu, X., Wang, B., Zhang, Q., Zhang, J. and Wang, S., 2023. The long-term trend of uterine fibroid burden in China from 1990 to 2019: A Joinpoint and Age–Period–Cohort study. Frontiers in Physiology, 14, p.1197658.

Lou, Z., Huang, Y., Li, S., Luo, Z., Li, C., Chu, K., Zhang, T., Song, P. and Zhou, J., 2023. Global, regional, and national time trends in incidence, prevalence, years lived with disability for uterine fibroids, 1990–2019: an age-period-cohort analysis for the global burden of disease 2019 study. BMC Public Health, 23(1), p.916.

Malekinejad, H. and Rezabakhsh, A., 2015. Hormones in dairy foods and their impact on public health-a narrative review article. Iranian journal of public health, 44(6), p.742.

McKenna, K.A. and Fogleman, C.D., 2021. Dysmenorrhea. American family physician, 104(2), pp.164-170.

Messina, M., 2016. Soy and health update: evaluation of the clinical and epidemiologic literature. Nutrients, 8(12), p.754.a

Mobeen, S. and Apostol, R., 2020. Ovarian cyst.

Mohammed, R.A., 2022. Diosmin for Treatment of Menorrhagia in Women Using Copper IUD. The Egyptian Journal of Hospital Medicine, 89(1), pp.5728-5732.

Nedresky, D. and Singh, G., 2019. Physiology, luteinizing hormone.

NHS, 2023. Ovarian Cyst: Causes. Available at https://www.nhs.uk/conditions/ovarian-cyst/causes/#:~:text=But%20sometimes%20a%20follicle%20does,symptoms%20such%20as%20pelvic%20pain.

Nowak, K., Ratajczak–Wrona, W., Górska, M. and Jabłońska, E., 2018. Parabens and their effects on the endocrine system. Molecular and cellular endocrinology, 474, pp.238-251.

Oduwole, O.O., Huhtaniemi, I.T. and Misrahi, M., 2021. The roles of luteinizing hormone, follicle-stimulating hormone and testosterone in spermatogenesis and folliculogenesis revisited.

International journal of molecular sciences, 22(23), p.12735.

Oregon State University, n.d. Indole-3-Carbinol. https://lpi.oregonstate.edu/mic/dietary-factors/phytochemicals/indole-3-carbinol

Oregon State University, n.d. Resveratrol. Oregon State University, https://lpi.oregonstate.edu/mic/dietary-factors/phytochemicals/resveratrol#:~:text=Resveratrol%20is%20found%20in%20grapes,in%20the%20skins%20(144).

Palter, S. and Olive, D., 2002. Reproductive physiology. Novak's Gynecology, ed. Berek, SJ (Philadelphia: Lippincott Williams & Wilkins, 2002), 159.

Patel, N., Chaudhari, K., Patel, D., Joshi, J., Patel Jr, N., Patel, D.J. and Joshi, J.S., 2023. High Intensity Focused Ultrasound Ablation of Uterine Fibroids: A Review. Cureus, 15(9).

Peterson, J., Dwyer, J., Adlercreutz, H., Scalbert, A., Jacques, P. and McCullough, M.L., 2010. Dietary lignans: physiology and potential for cardiovascular disease risk reduction. Nutrition reviews, 68(10), pp.571-603.

Pirtea, P., de Ziegler, D. and Ayoubi, J.M., 2023. Endometrial receptivity in adenomyosis and/or endometriosis. Fertility and Sterility.

Przygrodzka, E., Plewes, M.R. and Davis, J.S., 2021. Luteinizing hormone regulation of inter-organelle communication and fate of the corpus luteum.

International journal of molecular sciences, 22(18), p.9972.

Purwar, A. and Nagpure, S., 2022. Insulin resistance in polycystic ovarian syndrome. Cureus, 14(10).

Rahmadani, S. and Furqan, M., 2022. Backward Chaining Method for Diagnosis Disorders of Women's Menstrual Cycle. Jurnal Mantik, 6(3), pp.3137-3143.

Raja, M.H.R., Farooqui, N., Zuberi, N., Ashraf, M., Azhar, A., Baig, R., Badar, B. and Rehman, R., 2021. Endometriosis, infertility and MicroRNA's: A review. Journal of Gynecology Obstetrics and Human Reproduction, 50(9), p.102157.

Rocha-González, H.I., Ambriz-Tututi, M. and Granados-Soto, V., 2008. Resveratrol: a natural compound with pharmacological potential in neurodegenerative diseases. CNS neuroscience & therapeutics, 14(3), pp.234-247.

Rodríguez-García, C., Sánchez-Quesada, C., Toledo, E., Delgado-Rodríguez, M. and Gaforio, J.J., 2019. Naturally lignan-rich foods: A dietary tool for health promotion?. Molecules, 24(5), p.917.

Shah, M.Z.U.H. and Shrivastava, V.K., 2023. Ameliorative effects of quercetin on endocrine and metabolic abnormalities associated with experimentally induced polycystic ovary syndrome in mice. Comparative Clinical Pathology, pp.1-9.

Sharma, S. and Tripathi, A., 2022. Endometriosis: The Enigma That It Continues to Be.

Smolarz, B., Szyłło, K. and Romanowicz, H., 2021. Endometriosis: epidemiology, classification, pathogenesis, treatment and genetics (review of literature). International journal of molecular sciences, 22(19), p.10554.

Song, S.D., Acharya, K.D., Zhu, J.E., Deveney, C.M., Walther-Antonio, M.R., Tetel, M.J. and Chia, N., 2020. Daily vaginal microbiota fluctuations associated with natural hormonal cycle, contraceptives, diet, and exercise. MSphere, 5(4), pp.10-1128.

Spritzer, P.M., Marchesan, L.B., Santos, B.R. and Fighera, T.M., 2022. Hirsutism, normal androgens and diagnosis of PCOS. Diagnostics, 12(8), p.1922.

Starkman, E., 2021. What Are Phthalates? WebMD, https://www.webmd.com/a-to-z-guides/features/what-are-phthalates

Wang, J., Chen, B., Hu, F., Zou, X., Yu, H., Wang, J., He, H., Zhang, H. and Huang, W., 2017. Effect of hispolon from Phellinus lonicerinus (Agaricomycetes) on estrogen receptors, aromatase, and cyclooxygenase II in MCF-7 breast cancer cells. International Journal of Medicinal Mushrooms, 19(3).

WebMD, 2021. What to Know About Parabens. https://www.webmd.com/beauty/what-to-know-about-parabens

WebMD, 2022. Top Foods High in Estrogen. WebMD, https://www.webmd.com/diet/foods-high-in-estrogen

WHO, 2023a. Polycystic ovary syndrome. Key Facts. Available at https://www.who.int/news-room/fact-sheets/detail/polycystic-ovary-syndrome#:~:text=Polycystic%20ovary%20syndrome%20(PCOS)%20affects,a%20leading%20cause%20of%20infertility.

WHO, 2023b. Endometriosis. World Health Organization. Available at https://www.who.int/news-room/fact-sheets/detail/endometriosis#:~:text=Key%20facts,age%20women%20and%20girls%20globally.

Woldemeskel, M., 2022. Toxicologic pathology of the reproductive system. In Reproductive and developmental toxicology (pp. 1289-1321). Academic Press.

Xu, Y. and Qiao, J., 2022. Association of insulin resistance and elevated androgen levels with polycystic ovarian syndrome (PCOS): a review of literature. Journal of healthcare engineering, 2022.

Zhang, Y., Cao, H., Yu, Z., Peng, H.Y. and Zhang, C.J., 2013. Curcumin inhibits endometriosis endometrial cells by reducing estradiol production. Iranian journal of reproductive medicine, 11(5), p.415.

ABOUT THE AUTHOR

Zecaina N. N.

Is a firm believer in the concept of patient-centred healthcare and has therefore made it his life mission to empower individuals struggling with various medical complications through provision of healthcare knowledge. With this mission, he hopes to help people recover from their conditions in a cost-effective, home-based, and efficient manner.

BOOKS BY THIS AUTHOR

Fighting Depressive Illness And Suicidal Thoughts: First-Hand Experience Of Treating And Healing From Depression

Are you tired of people telling you, "avoid thinking about it," when you open up about struggling with the depressive illness in order to get help? Are you exhausted with hearing, "don't do it; life is precious," as the solution to suicidal thoughts?

Well, I promise to not try selling you the same story as the answer to treating depression.

Why? Because, I have been there and I know how it feels! When you are trying to find a depression cure, not thinking about it is always the answer that you get first. But, the truth of the matter is - it doesn't work in the slightest bit.

I'm also not going to sell you hot air in the name of self-empowerment. I'm not here to tell you, "You're much stronger than you think," "If you set your mind you can overcome," or, "You just have to fight harder."

Why? Same reason - I've been there, and I know how it feels. When you're struggling with the depressive illness and suicidal thoughts, you usually are at your weakest point. You basically have no willpower to pushback or fight. And when somebody tries to tell you, "You can beat this," you right away know that you don't have the power to do it. I mean, if you had the strength of healing from depression on your own through psychological empowerment, you wouldn't be seeking help in the first place, right?

So, what is this book about?

Well, for starters, I share my personal experience of how I struggled with the depressive illness and suicidal thoughts. I do so with hope that my story is going to remind you that you're not alone as you struggle with the depressive illness and suicidal thoughts.

Then, I tell you how to overcome depression based on my personal experience. And since I'm a believer in natural remedies and homemade remedies, my solution of treating and healing from depression won't be one that adds more money to the pockets of big pharma.

The Obesity Textbook Of How Lose Weight Like Crazy - A Weight Loss Memoir With A

Guideline To Cut Fat And Shed Weight Fast

There are tons of books out there that promise to show you the secrets of how to lose weight like crazy. And, you've most probably read a bunch of them. So, what is different about this book?

Well, for starters, it is a weight loss memoir! Yes, it is written by someone that was formerly obese.

Thus, it's not just another pathetic attempt to cramp words together in the name of "an obesity textbook" so as to milk money from your problems. This obesity textbook offers the real experience of how I managed to cut fat and shed weight fast.

Rather than sell you hot air about obese weight loss, this obesity textbook gives you the scientifically proven method of how to lose weight like crazy - it has some mathematical formulas and calculations.

But, enough of tooting my own horn! Time for you to read my weight loss memoir, practice its guidelines, and see if you won't cut fat and shed weight fast.

Trauma Focused Cbt For Children And Adolescents: The Practical Guide For Healing Developmental Trauma And Coming Out Of Ptsd

No matter how strong you are; the process of healing developmental trauma can be very challenging. Just when you think you are finally making some progress - you end up backsliding into the pit. And the worst part is that it happens over and over.

But, don't worry! This book is the stable and reliable solution you need for coming out of PTSD. And, in case you're wondering why I'm so sure it's going to work for you; that's where I'm headed next.

Cognitive Behavioral Therapy (CBT) is increasingly gaining popularity within the field of psychology as a dependable and effective approach for treating various mental health issues. Whether it is depression, anxiety, bipolar disorder, post-traumatic stress disorder (PTSD), or schizophrenia; CBT always has a way out!

So, if you focused on healing developmental trauma, why not do it with one of the most scientifically proven and psychologically accepted methods?

Don't know how to go about it? That's where this book - Trauma focused CBT for children and adolescents: The practical guide for healing developmental trauma and coming out of PTSD - comes in handy.

www.ingramcontent.com/pod-product-compliance
Lightning Source LLC
Chambersburg PA
CBHW050850260726
48660CB00006B/2543